THE FACTS ABOUT THE
MENOPAUSE

Other Books in the Need2Know Series

A full list of books can be obtained from
Need2Know, 1-2 Wainman Road, Woodston, Peterborough PE2 7BU

Help Yourself to a Job
Step by step into work
Jackie Lewis

Buying a House
Ease the path to your new front door
John Docker

Stretch your Money
Get more for your £££'s
Michael Herschell

Make the Most of Retirement
Live your new life to the full
Mike Mogano

Make the Most of Being a Carer
A practical guide to lightening the load
Ann Whitfield

Breaking Up
Live your new life to the full
Chris West

Successful Writing
The beginner's guide to selling your work
Teresa McCuaig

Superwoman
A practical guide for working mothers
Marion Jayawardene

Work for yourself and Win
A practical guide to successful
self-employment
Ian Gretton

The Expatriate Experience
A practical guide to successful relocation
Bobby Meyer

Forget the Fear of Food
A positive approach to healthy eating
Dr Christine Fenn Accredited Nutritionist

You and your Tenancy
A helpful guide to feeling at home
Sue Dyson

Improving your Lifestyle
Live a more satisfying life
Mike Mogano

Safe as Houses
Security and safety in the home
Gordon Wells

The World's your Oyster
Education and training for adults
Polly Bird

Everything you Need2Know About Sex
The A-Z Guide to Increase your Knowledge
Anne Johnson

Travel Without Tears
An Essential Guide to Happy Family
Holidays
Marion Jayawardene

Prime Time Mothers
A Positive Approach to Delayed Maternity
Lyn Cartner

Parenting Teenagers
Make the Most of this Unique Relationship
Polly Bird

Planning your Wedding
A Step by Step Guide to the Happy Day
Niamh O'Kiersey

Make a Success of Family Life
A Guide to Getting Along
Michael Herschell

Coping With Bereavement
Julie Armstrong-Colton

Get What You Pay For
A Guide to Consumer Rights
Gordon Wells

Take a Career Break
Bringing Up Children Without Giving Up
Your Future
Astrid Stevens

Forthcoming books in 1997 series
(Working titles only)

Fertility Problems
Dr Phyllis Mortimer

Learning Difficulties
Maria Chivers

Beating Stress
Nick Daws

Parents Guide to Drugs
Judy Mackie

**Getting the Best out of Education for
your Children**
David Abbott

Successful Relationships for Singles
Sheila O'Connor

Your Child Starting Primary School
Lyn Cartner

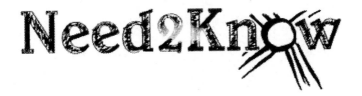

THE FACTS ABOUT THE MENOPAUSE

Coping Before, During and After

Elliot Philipp

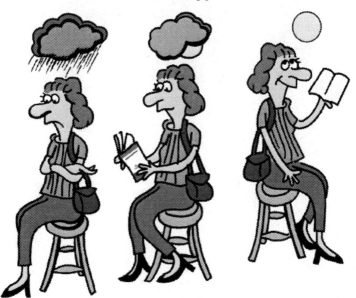

Need2Know

© Elliot Philipp 1996
ISBN 1 86144 022 7

First published November 1996

First published by Need2Know, 1-2 Wainman Road,
Woodston, Peterborough, Cambridgeshire PE2 7BU
Tel 01733 390801 Fax 01733 230751

All rights reserved
Edited by Kerrie Pateman
Design by Spencer Hart
Typesetting by Forward Press Ltd

Contents

Introduction

What the Menopause is

The menopause is that period in a woman's life that marks the end of her ability to have children. The reproductive years last from the ages of about 15 to 45 on average. One or perhaps two eggs each month are released from an ovary. These eggs are capable of being fertilised and the woman may be capable of having children as a result. Fertility, which means her chances of getting pregnant and delivering a baby, diminish rapidly after the age of 40, partly because the number of eggs produced in the ovaries declines and partly because the eggs are of poorer quality and do not become easily fertilised no matter how good the partner's semen is.

The average age of the menopause in the United Kingdom is about 51, but the menopause can quite normally occur at any time between the ages of 46 and 56. Twenty years ago girls were having their first periods earlier and women their last periods later than they did forty or fifty years ago. Reproductive life is therefore lasting longer; but the trend to start reproductive life earlier has now stopped.

A woman is menopausal *one year after* her last period. Although by definition the menopause is the time of the last period; it is difficult to know at the time that it is the last period as another may still come. Also many women's periods become spaced out so that instead of having a period regularly every month, she may only have one every two or three months or even six months. They become quite irregular. That is why a woman is not really menopausal until a year after her last period. If a woman has her last period at the age of 35 or earlier, she has suffered a 'premature menopause'. The youngest patient I have had with a premature menopause was only 19. That was terribly early.

There are three stages to the menopause. The first is *pre-menopausal*, ie before the menopause when the hormones are changing their pattern of activity. The second stage is the *menopause* itself when finally the last period has occurred, and the third is the *post-menopausal* stage, when a woman is certain that she has had her last period and can safely stop contraceptive methods because the risk of her getting pregnant has disappeared. Surprises rarely occur but although women at this time are much less fertile, a few become pregnant within the year after the last period. An odd egg that has been left behind can be released from an ovary within this year - so it is better to be careful than to have a surprise.

A woman's life can be divided into three phases:
- ✿ prepubertal
- ✿ reproductive age
- ✿ post-menopausal (for many this is 'the third and best stage of life')

The years around the menopause are the *peri-menopausal* years. Others call it the *climacteric* from the Greek word 'Klimakter' which means 'rung of a ladder'. About ten million women in the UK are going through the menopause or have gone through it. Many of these women find these are very good years. They are settled with their partners; they are freed of some of their domestic responsibilities; they may, or may not, have retired from work; so they can either concentrate more on their hobbies or take up new occupations. Some welcome taking on new responsibilities. Some of our most successful women in politics, in local councils and in Parliament, and some of the leaders in industry, are menopausal or post-menopausal ladies. In many ways they are much freer than ever before. Some have been able to take up new professions and new occupations because they have never previously had the opportunity to do these things. What is more the numbers are being added to as women's health improves, and people live longer.

This is not to say that the menopause is all a bed of roses for everybody. Few women suffer from every complaint, but most women in a minor way at least, do have one or more of the following rather unpleasant symptoms before they are completely through the menopausal years. This is the list in order of frequency, but not in order of severity:

✪ Irritability, can affect about 90% of all women going through the menopause
✪ Lethargy, affects about 80%
✪ Depression, affects 50%
✪ Hot flushes and night sweats affect about 70%
✪ Mild headaches are not uncommon at this age
✪ Forgetfulness, which also tends to affect men in later years
✪ Some weight gain occurs if women 'let go' and do not cut down on their food intake which they have to do to take account of less energy being used up
✪ Most women do not need to sleep quite so long and think they are suffering from insomnia
✪ A few joint pains are common
✪ Some women do have palpitations and some have crying spells
✪ Constipation affects a few
✪ Sometimes the very last periods can be painful
✪ As for their sex drive most women find to their surprise that it has gone up but for about 20% it goes down

The list on the previous page has been compiled from questionnaires completed by patients in menopause clinics.

This rather daunting list is virtually self limiting without treatment. For some it does continue for a long time and a few of the symptoms quite often last for four or five years - never for more than ten years. All are treatable.

Just a word about hot flushes which affect about three quarters of all women at some time in the menopausal years. These usually begin in the face, the neck, the head or the chest, and parts of the hands. Each flush involves a reddening of the skin which can last anything from a few seconds to half an hour or so. We do not know exactly why they occur, but it may be that higher levels of FSH or LH somehow act on the blood vessels under the skin. More about these hormones and of the symptoms of the menopause will be detailed later.

Lethargy, which is quite common, means that some women should take things a little easier. Copying the late Winston Churchill's habit of having a doze in the middle of the afternoon after which he spent the rest of the day with renewed energy can be the best way for you to cope with this very common symptom.

Irritability is perhaps the most

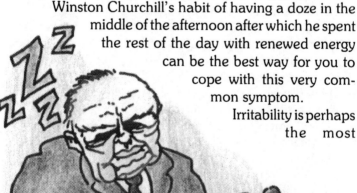

common of all the disturbances and is much easier to bear for those around the irritable lady if they know that it is 'the change'.

The need for medical checks

It is very important indeed to realise that some of the symptoms mentioned above may be due to real illnesses or real character changes. You may therefore need a doctor to investigate them. Anyhow it is recommended that all women should have fairly regular check-ups including smear tests and I am sure that no woman should go on to HRT (Hormone Replacement Therapy) without a proper assessment by her doctor. If you think any symptom you have is worrying, do see your doctor. Do not say to yourself 'it's my time of life'. It is not likely to be just that, you may all too easily have a disturbance that can easily be treated. Doctors are now very used to being consulted by women going through the menopause - and they should be.

1

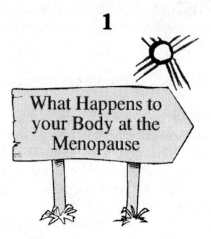

The clock turns back a little
The other end, the start of reproductive life
How do doctors tell that their patients are menopausal?

This chapter is a little technical. It can be skipped at the first reading but you may want to come back to it later.

The clock turns back a little

The menopause is the time when periods (mensis = monthly) stop. This change usually starts by the periods becoming more spaced out; or they become lighter in quantity, or with some women they just stop, may be quite suddenly. All this is normal.

Sometimes things that are not quite normal happen. The periods may become heavier. They may become more frequent. They may even become painful. These are not normal happenings and if they carry on for more than a few months they certainly should be investigated by a doctor and probably by a specialist.

Why does the lessening of the blood flow occur? The

answer is because the store of eggs in the ovaries has become used up.

The other end, the start, of reproductive life

It is easier to understand what happens at the menopause if we realise that what is going on is a partial reversal of what happened at the other end of reproductive life. In the years before puberty from the age of about 10 onwards, changes are starting which take about three years to develop fully. From the age of about 10 to 13 breasts start to bud and small quantities of hair appear over the pubis and under the armpits. Periods start a little later and their start is called the 'menarche'. This term which is used by doctors is made up from the Latin word 'mensis' (month) and a Greek word 'arche' (the beginning). The menarche normally occurs somewhere between 10 to 16 years of age. For this to happen the uterus and the vagina have enlarged and at the beginning the girl starts what is called a 'growth spurt'. She goes on growing in height quite rapidly for another three or four years after her first period. At puberty or the menarche the uterus under the influence of hormones has developed a thickish lining. Not only does the girl grow taller but also stronger as her muscles and her bones grow and much calcium and other substances including minerals are deposited in the bones; providing she takes normal quantities of exercise and eats well.

All this happens because of the action of different groups of hormones. Understanding the way these hormones come into play makes it easier for us to understand how when the menopause comes thirty to forty years later the reversal takes place.

There is an organ called the hypothalamus in the lower part of the brain. It releases chemicals called 'releasing factors'. Severe emotional upsets and abnormal eating habits such as anorexia, and excessive physical exercise can disturb the proper functioning of the hypothalamus which is rather like a very sophisticated calendar clock that controls when periods start and stop, among other things. The hypothalamus in girls with anorexia stops putting out releasing factors to control and start the menstrual cycle. That is a very protective mechanism because monthly periods would be very damaging to girls who in any case are not getting enough iron from their food.

The releasing hormones from the hypothalamus influence many other hormone producing organs in the body, but for our purposes the most important one that is influenced to secrete hormones is the anterior pituitary gland. This is situated just below the hypothalamus in the base of the skull (see Fig 1). The two hormones are the follicle stimulating hormone (FSH) and the luteinizing hormone (LH). FSH and LH in their turn act on the ovaries.

The two *ovaries* are situated in the pelvis on each side

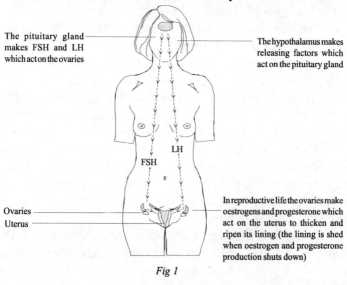

The pituitary gland makes FSH and LH which act on the ovaries

The hypothalamus makes releasing factors which act on the pituitary gland

LH

FSH

Ovaries
Uterus

In reproductive life the ovaries make oestrogens and progesterone which act on the uterus to thicken and ripen its lining (the lining is shed when oestrogen and progesterone production shuts down)

Fig 1

of the uterus. When a girl is born each ovary contains about a half to one million cells which could in theory ripen into eggs, but only about 400 do during reproductive life, and none before or after. Many just die off before puberty so that there are only about 100,000 left, but still that leaves a large reserve.

As only one of these primitive eggs will develop into a ripe egg to be released in the middle of each menstrual cycle - about 14 days after the period has started - there is considerable wastage because the whole 100,000 are used up by the time of the menopause. By the age of 45 there are perhaps only a few hundred left and they are not of as good quality as those that were released at the age of 25. In a young woman the follicle stimulating hormone (FSH) of the pituitary makes one follicle, or perhaps two follicles in an ovary mature, so that on about the 14th day of the cycle one ovary releases an egg or rarely two. Luteinising hormone (LH) from the pituitary acts to make the lining of the burst follicle put down some yellow tissue (corpus luteum). The two ovaries probably take it in turn to ripen and release an egg each month.

The ovary, under the influence of FSH, makes oestrogens, and under the influence of LH it makes progesterone. These hormones produced by the ovaries are all important for reproductive life.

Oestrogens act in several ways. They make the lining of the womb which after a period has become very thin, thicken up again. They also send messages by a 'feedback' process to the pituitary gland (see Fig 2) to slow down the production of FSH. They are also concerned with the development of the breasts.

Progesterone acts in a different way. It makes the lining of the womb which has thickened take on a more complicated pattern. This pattern allows small pits to develop in the lining of the womb and it is in one of these that a fertilised egg can lodge, and take hold and start a

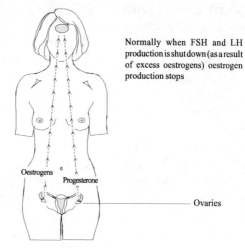

Normally when FSH and LH production is shut down (as a result of excess oestrogens) oestrogen production stops

When the oestrogens and progesterone reach high levels in the blood a 'feedback' message is sent out to the pituitary to tell it to stop FSH and LH production temporarily

Oestrogens

Progesterone

Ovaries

At the menopause because no oestrogens and progesterone reach the pituitary to tell it to shut down FSH and LH production, FSH increases greatly.

Fig 2 The feedback mechanism

pregnancy. Progesterone also acts on the breasts so that oestrogen and progesterone together may make the breasts feel tense (as in pre-menstrual tension).

Periods are really the tears of a disappointed womb. Each month it prepares to receive a fertilised egg and when no egg is deposited in it, which is invariably the case if fertilisation has not taken place, the process shuts down for that month. Because of the *feed-back* mechanism of oestrogens from the ovary acting on the pituitary gland, FSH production is temporarily stopped and progesterone feed-back stops LH production in the pituitary for a few days. When the uterus is deprived of oestrogens and progesterone it gets rid of most but not all the thickness of the lining of the womb. This redundant tissue is washed away by blood that flows from small arteries in the inner surface of the womb. This is a period. Normally a period lasts from three to seven days (see glossary).

The hypothalamus then takes over again the job of sending out releasing hormones to start the whole cycle over again so that every 28 days or so the whole sequence is repeated. Bone is deposited in the skeleton quite rapidly for the next three years after the first period, providing the young woman takes sufficient exercise. The pull of muscles during exercise helps bone to grow. Calcium and other minerals are needed to give the bones strength and they are deposited in greater quantities in adolescence, which are the years following the menarche, than at any other time.

So what happens in the menopause when the complicated cycle that had been initiated 30 years or so earlier, starts to be reversed? Well, the most important thing is that as all the eggs are used up there is nothing left to burst out of the follicle which has enlarged under FSH stimulus. In fact there are also very few follicles left. The follicle cannot produce oestrogens and so their levels in the blood go down as does the level of progesterone. Because there is no feed-back of the oestrogens to the pituitary it still goes on making FSH in an uninhibited way and this can be detected by measuring the FSH in the blood.

We think that it is the overproduction of FSH which is not damped down by the feed-back from the ovary that leads to most of the symptoms of the menopause including the hot flushes. Over production of FSH and LH are not beneficial. How can we stop it? Quite simply by giving hormones particularly oestrogens which we know will go to the pituitary and stop it producing excess FSH and LH.

What were the changes that were so noticeable in the young woman at puberty? Firstly enlargement of the breasts. Once breasts have developed they will not disappear, even if oestrogens are withdrawn, but some breasts do lose some of their firmness at the menopause, as may other tissues. The muscles of the abdomen can slacken off a little if they are not kept in tone by good exercise and for some unknown reason there is also a tendency for some fat to be put down in undesirable places such as the hips and the middle of the abdomen.

Of course because there are no eggs the risk of pregnancy has gone. One good result of stopping periods is that the monthly small drain on the iron reserves of the body also stops. There is no more risk of anaemia from heavy periods.

Many women feel a new burst of energy at the menopause, probably because they are less anaemic and with the cessation of the 'curse' of the periods they don't have to worry about being pregnant. If they were a little anaemic the haemoglobin, the important chemical in the blood to take oxygen around increases in quantity. No wonder that many women have new bursts of energy at the menopause. These sometimes reveal themselves in unexpected ways such as an increase in *libido*, the wish to make love. This happens particularly if she has a partner who can participate in this new energy and accompany her to her new interests. He may very well be delighted with her new sexual energy and they should use this increased libido because regular sex is good for health in itself and seems to keep up the production of other hormones needed in a healthy body. Some women unfortunately find their libido has gone down and want to have it restored though only about 20% of women find this but hormones prescribed and taken in the right way will put that right.

You cannot buy hormones over the counter. Hormone replacement therapy (HRT) has to be prescribed by a doctor. If it is not absolutely obvious that you are in the menopause the doctor may order some tests to confirm that you are either going through the menopause or have completed it.

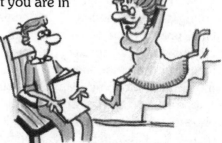

How do doctors tell that their patients are menopausal?

Firstly they listen to what the woman is telling them and examine the patient carefully because they should have a record of the woman's state of health before she starts HRT. Normally at this visit to decide on HRT the weight is noted, urine is tested, the breasts are carefully examined, blood pressure taken and a smear test carried out. At the same time the doctor performs a thorough pelvic examination to make sure that there are no abnormalities there such as fibroids in the uterus or cysts in the ovaries. Many doctors now arrange a routine mammogram at this stage.

But we live in a scientific age and a doctor may still want to confirm that his patient is menopausal. He does this most accurately by taking blood from a vein in the arm and sending it to the laboratory where a test is made for the level of oestrogens (which would have gone down) and follicle stimulating hormone, which as explained before, will have gone up. If this has happened and he gets a low oestrogen and a high FSH reading he knows he is dealing with a menopausal lady. If you object to having blood taken there is a cheaper, easier test which is called 'the Progestogen Challenge Test'. Normally the uterus does not bleed as a result of being treated with progestogens in tablet form unless its lining has become ripened and thickened with oestrogens. We have seen that the absence or very low level of oestrogens is the hall mark of the menopause. If a woman is given Progestogens daily for ten days and does not bleed within a few days after stopping the tablets it means that the lining of the womb has not thickened because there is no oestrogen present. So the negative progestogen bleeding test is good evidence that the menopause has arrived.

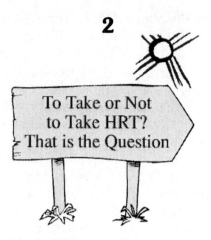

2

To Take or Not
to Take HRT?
That is the Question

Who should take HRT and be likely to benefit greatly?
The changes in the breasts on HRT
Those who should take HRT
What about the remaining 45%, who perhaps should not take HRT?
HRT, the menopause and breast cancer

Who should take HRT and be likely to benefit greatly?

I do not believe that every woman must take HRT. This chapter explains how you can decide whether HRT is for you or not. I do believe that the majority of women will benefit from it if they take it for about five years or may be a little longer. Women doctors in the United Kingdom have decided what to do for themselves.

There was an article in the British Medical Journal in November 1995 about a sample of women doctors in the UK who had qualified and registered in the years 1952 and 1976.

Out of 1000 women doctors whose names were selected at random and who were between 43 and 65 years of age, 45% had used HRT at some time or other. As most of those still menstruating were not using it the researchers took them out; so that when they only counted doctors who were past the age at which they had menstruated - ie were really menopausal, they found that 55% had used HRT at some time or other. Some doctors dropped out, but about 70% of those who had started HRT were continuing it 5 years later, and over 50% ten years later. We see that over half of all women doctors believe that HRT is good for them and they are women who really should know.

The changes in the breasts on HRT

A little lumpiness or being able to feel small nodules in the breast is common before the menopause. This unevenness becomes less marked after the menopause if HRT is not being taken. If it is being taken then the unevenness in the breasts returns as the hormones go through the body to the breasts. If a woman feels a *definite* lump - no matter how small - she should quickly go to her general practitioner to have a check. If little nodules however just come and go, a woman should make a note of these changes because they may not be serious.

Those who should take HRT

Women who have had a hysterectomy and especially those who have had the operation before the normal age of the menopause really should seriously consider taking

HRT. If the surgeon has removed both ovaries at the time of the hysterectomy the likelihood of developing symptoms early is much greater. Most gynaecologists recommend nearly all hysterectomized patients to take HRT and some go so far as to put an implant in at the time of the hysterectomy to make quite sure that their patients are having HRT. Women who have had a hysterectomy do not need to take Progestogens which are Progesterone like substances. They are at some advantage because without progesterone they are a little less likely to develop side effects such as symptoms of pre-menstrual tension (PMT).

Once you have decided to take HRT you should continue it, and not be put off too quickly by any side effects you may have. The most common side effects are occasional feelings of nausea, but no actual sickness, and very commonly particularly if you are having progestogens as well, tenderness of the breasts, sensitivity of the nipples and leg cramps. All these symptoms disappear by themselves after a few months either continuing with the first preparation you have tried, or else disappear when you try a different preparation.

There are so many on the market that it is quite advisable to swap around until you find the one that suits you best (see chapter 4). The side effects of HRT, which will certainly go, are a small price to pay for the relief of the symptoms of the menopause - the flushes, the hot sweats and so on, and the long term troubles of osteoporosis. HRT takes a little time to act. With some patients the effect is very rapid, but it can take up to three months for the flushes and the night sweats to be improved, and up to six months for the bladder control and some of the vaginal dryness and tightness to go, and may be even a year for depression to disappear. But they can be prevented if HRT is taken soon enough.

Any woman who has had a bone scan which shows that the bones are less dense than they should be, should certainly take HRT or Fosamax (see Chapter 7) in order to avoid fractured bones which can be real killers in older women. HRT in your fifties can protect your bones in your seventies.

What about the remaining 45%, who perhaps should not take HRT?

The fervid advocates of HRT think that there are very few women who will not benefit but I am not one of those because:

✿ I do not like the idea of persuading anybody to do anything she does not want to do. Women should not take HRT if they do not want to. I see all too many women who feel they have to take HRT just to be in the swing of things. This is no more necessary than having to follow the current fashion for clothing or for hairstyle. Some women's gut feelings tell them what is good for them. I often hear women say 'I know my body very well, and I know what it wants'. I am not quite sure that anybody knows their body very well, because the human body is such a complicated structure that no one is able to know everything about it. But, 'I know what it wants' surely means 'I know what I want or do not want', and that is another matter. So, nobody should be forced to do anything or take anything they really do not want to. I have always said to my students 'never force anything on anybody unless it is absolutely essential'. By essential I mean something like removing a cancerous lump or treating it with chemotherapy or radiotherapy. So, I suggest you should not be forced to take hormones if you do not want to, unless there is a definite indication for them such as osteoporosis or a tendency to osteoporosis has been diagnosed. In that case by taking hormones you will avoid fractured bones later

✿ The next and perhaps biggest category of women who should not be taking HRT are those who do not need it. This applies particularly to women who are already on the pill which delivers them more than enough hormones and can be continued until the age of 52 to 53

✿ As is described in another chapter (page 21) doctors can tell quite scientifically whether a woman is likely to benefit from taking hormones by estimating the FSH and the oestrogen levels in the blood. I do not think you should take HRT because you have reached the age when your friends start it. There are big differences in the ages at which different women start their menopause and their need for HRT. If your body is behaving perfectly normally and you are having no symptoms and your hormone levels are normal, then you do not need HRT and I cannot see that there is any point in taking it

✿ Another group of women who should not take HRT are those with fibroids in the uterus. HRT makes fibroids grow. If you really feel you must take HRT then you will have to have your fibroids removed either by the operation to destroy them with laser or by having them shelled out which is a bigger procedure or by having a hysterectomy. I do not think having a hysterectomy just to be able to take HRT is a very clever thing although there are hundreds of thousands of women in the United States who do have this operation in order to allow them to take HRT, even if they have not really got a real indication for hysterectomy such as fibroids

✿ The next category of women who should not be on HRT is those having heavy periods. It is alright to start HRT once the periods start diminishing

✿ I think women with cystic breasts or lumpy breasts should also not take HRT unless their symptoms of the menopause are debilitating, and they have had either a mammogram or an ultrasound scan which shows that the breasts are completely normal. Some HRT makes breasts that are already cystic more so

HRT, The Menopause and Breast Cancer

In spite of the many millions of pounds that have been spent on research, doctors still do not know the cause or causes of cancer of the breast. Recently a gene has been discovered in parts of cells in the body (the chromosomes) which may be responsible in some families with a tendency for women in those families to develop cancer of the breast in succeeding generations. Unfortunately, cancer of the breast is a very common disease.

Certain conditions seem to favour the development of cancer in other organs. Unopposed oestrogens will increase the likelihood of a woman with a womb developing cancer of the lining of the womb. Unprotected exposure to the sun will increase the likelihood of sunbathers developing a cancer of the skin. Exposure to high doses of radiation is also known to increase the likelihood of cancer of the blood. But, we do not know whether hormones, and in particular oestrogens, favour the development of breast cancer.

What is fairly certain is that if a woman has been on HRT for ten to fifteen years her risk of developing cancer of the breast seems to be increased by about one third. This means that if the medical histories of 100,000 women who have never taken HRT at all were examined it would be found that about 'x' number have developed cancer of the breast. If the medical histories of 100,000 women who have taken HRT for more than 10 years are examined, then 'x plus one third of x' number of women will have developed cancer of the breast. But if true, doctors do not know what it is in the HRT that has done that.

If you take HRT for only five years the chances of developing cancer of the breast are not increased at all.

A number of eminent doctors met at the Royal Society of Medicine in May 1994 to discuss HRT and breast cancer. They concluded that whether to recommend HRT or not to women with a risk of developing cancer of the breast posed a serious ethical dilemma for them.

Professor Michael Baum, probably our greatest expert on the subject, thinks that doctors will really only know what to recommend from this point of view after they have carried out randomised control trials, which means giving very large numbers of women HRT and keeping a close watch on them and keeping an equally close watch on an equally large number of women who are not taking HRT. He told me very recently that we would have to wait ten years to see what the outcome of these trials was going to be. Meanwhile this may deprive large numbers of women of the real benefits of HRT, without definite proof that they are going to be saved from getting cancer of the breast. In fact some of them will anyway, but more will die of heart attacks and from the effects of osteoporosis than would have died from cancer of the breast.

If a woman has been diagnosed as having a small cancerous lump in her breast, has had it removed successfully and has been free of cancer for some years, can she safely take HRT? We really do not know. The doctors in the May 1994 conference said that it was a scandal that they could not give an answer.

So what are you to do? We do know that women in certain categories are much less likely to develop cancer of the breast. These are women who have had a late menarche followed by an early pregnancy, followed by breast feeding for more than three months, and followed by another pregnancy. If they then have developed an early menopause either naturally or by having their ovaries removed their chances of developing cancer of the breast are much diminished.

Just one hundred years ago a doctor George Beatson found that when he had removed both ovaries from a woman who had advanced cancer of the breast, the cancer got smaller. He had given her an early menopause. So if you have the favourable factors of a late menarche, followed by the birth of two or more children whom you have breast fed and have an early menopause, you are considerably safer from the point of developing cancer of the breast than others. What should women with a strong family history of cancer of the breast do about HRT? Doctors really do not know. For my part I am at present very hesitant to prescribe HRT for these women, or if I do I prescribe it only for a year or two. There is a way out. Tamoxifen is a drug which has both oestrogen-like effects and effects that are against oestrogen. This is peculiar but Tamoxifen taken for a few years is a very good form of HRT for women who have already developed cancer of the breast. It even helps to prevent bone loss.

By and large I think it is safer for my patients who have a greater risk of cancer of the breast not to take HRT - *but* if their symptoms of the menopause are great I would give them relief from those symptoms by prescribing HRT for just a few years.

Women with a family history of cancer of the breast should probably avoid HRT. If a woman's mother and sister or mother and grandmother have had or worse still died from cancer of the breast there may be a family (genetic) disposition towards this disease and it is just possible, though by no means certain that taking oestrogens may turn that disposition into fact. If you do take HRT you need to have very frequent check-ups, which your doctor may decide should include regular mammograms.

Women who have had jaundice (hepatitis) should be screened to see whether they can tolerate HRT. Some women who have had jaundice in the past can take it, and others can not, and it may require a specialist to make the decision.

A woman should not think she is menopausal because she has missed a period or two and ask for HRT if she does not have a firm diagnosis of the menopause. The explanation may be that she is pregnant which is not an indication, definitely not, for taking HRT.

Some women who suffer from migraine headaches will benefit from HRT but others will not. You and your doctor have to decide whether your migraine means you should not be on HRT.

Some rare deafnesses and what is called 'otosclerosis' can be a contraindication to taking HRT.

If you get side effects from HRT you do not necessarily have to stop it. Usually a change to a different preparation is all that is necessary.

3

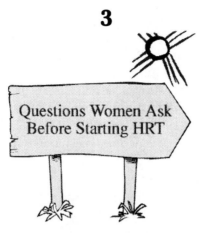

Questions Women Ask Before Starting HRT

Will I get cancer?
Will I put on weight?
Will I become less sexually active?
Will HRT cure the menopause?
Is HRT likely to give me a heart condition?

Will I get cancer?

There have been so many scare stories about women getting cancer because of HRT that it is very important to deal with this in an informed way. Firstly, cancer does not attack a *person*. It can attack specific *organs* in the body. In women cancer of the breast is common and so is cancer of the womb. In men cancer of the prostate is common. There are literally hundreds of different cancers that can affect different organs in different people at different ages. For instance skin cancers affect those who expose their skin to too much sunlight. Some kidney cancers affect young children.

What is a cancer?

Cancer occurs when cells in one part of the body start multiplying out of control. All cells normally multiply to take the place of old ones that have died or have been shed by say, something rubbing on the skin. In cancers the organs attacked cannot get rid of old worn-out cells as quickly as they make new ones and it is the excess of new ones growing in an uncontrolled way that causes the cancer.

Some cancers need hormones in order to grow. Cancer of the body of the womb for instance may grow when there is an unbalanced amount of oestrogen hormones acting on the lining of the womb. Cancer of the breast similarly has some slight dependency on hormones. Cancer of the neck of the womb we now know is more likely to be sexually transmitted than dependent on hormones. The only two organs that really concern us in connection with HRT are the breast and the body of the womb. It is certain that if a woman who has a womb (uterus) takes unopposed oestrogens (see pages 39-40) the lining of the womb will thicken right up and if it is not shed by regular bleeding can develop a cancer. That is why women who have not had their womb removed at hysterectomy are advised to take combined pills or at any rate progesterone to cause shedding of the lining of the womb. Combined oestrogen and progestogen treatment is a good prevention of cancer of the lining of the womb.

Cancer of the breast does occur more frequently in women on HRT. But the increase in numbers is small. Women can certainly develop cancer of the breast without taking hormones, but the likelihood of this developing if you take hormones is increased by just one third or less, and only in women who have been on HRT for more than

10 years. So, if a hundred women from the age of sixty who are not taking HRT develop cancer of the breast, then at the same age one hundred and thirty women on HRT may develop the cancer. If you take HRT for only five years there is no increased risk. You are not more likely to die younger because of the cancer of the breast if you are taking HRT, as your life will be very much prolonged because of the protective effects of HRT on the heart and on the brain preventing heart attacks and strokes.

In any case if you are on HRT you should have regular examinations which should include careful examinations of the breast by a doctor and cervical smears taken by a doctor or a nurse. Many doctors carry out mammograms which are x-rays of the breasts and which with the new low dose x-ray machines do *not* increase the likelihood of cancer.

Will I put on weight?

This is the second most frequently asked question when women discuss HRT. Yes, you possibly will because you will be feeling so much better that your appetite will increase and you will be less depressed. The only answer if you are putting on weight is to take more exercise to burn off the extra calories you are eating, or to cut down on what you eat. There is no need to put yourself on a diet because you are taking HRT. But, avoid second helpings, fatty foods, and sugar-containing foods like jams and marmalade. Marmalade is 50% sugar and very fattening, and so are many jams.

If I become more sexually active will my partner be able to keep up?

Every couple is different. Most men are simply delighted when their partner shows an extra interest in sex and take it as a compliment, and so it is. But some women have to look after their partners' health in some circumstances. For instance if your partner has angina it is wise not to stimulate him to perform too often. But if he wants to do it and you do, you can try to make it less physically demanding for him by having intercourse side by side or with you on top, if you like that. That saves him some effort because it is the physical exercise as well as the act of ejaculation that may occasionally put a strain on a man who is not absolutely fit. If he is working very hard during the week perhaps you might try to keep your sex to the weekends or times when he is needing to use less energy at his work. If you have been partners for a long time you will have developed a good enough relationship for him and you to talk it over together. Sadly, slightly older men who are married to women in their fifties are beginning to lose some but by no means all of their sex drive. Men having sex with their regular partners seldom have heart attacks then, but secret sex that a man may feel guilty about is bad for his heart. Happy sex with a regular partner is very good for both, not only from the point of view of morale but of health too.

Will I become less sexually active?

Definitely not. Most women find that because their hormone balance has come back to what it was before the menopause HRT hardly ever lowers their sex drive. It tends to raise it especially if dryness in the vagina is countered by the hormones.

If however, the vagina has become rather narrow because it has not been used much, it may need stretching, either by the fingers or by regular intercourse using a lubricant.

What do I have to do about contraception now since I am taking the same hormones that are found in the pill?

If you are on the pill just continue. The pill does contain much more in the way of hormones than HRT and it should not be taken for long after the menopause. The lower doses, in HRT are safer. On the other hand the lower doses in HRT are not sufficient to allow you to avoid contraception until at least a year after the end of the menopause, so you should still carry on with your usual contraceptive method. HRT is *not* a contraceptive because the hormone doses in it are too small to act as such.

Will HRT cure the menopause?

The menopause is not an illness and therefore HRT will not cure it. The menopause is a rebalancing of hormones and if they are not correctly balanced HRT will put that right.

Will I become hairy?

No. Female sex hormones do not make anybody hairy

but a few women at the menopause do develop stray hairs on the face and occasionally on the nipples because of a faulty balance of hormones. HRT will do little about that once it has happened but it can avoid it or prevent it happening if taken soon enough.

Will my vagina become inflamed?

No. HRT will not cause vaginitis (an inflamed infected vagina) but the increased sex activity if the vagina has been allowed to become narrow may result in some irritation. Beware of a new partner you may have found because of your need for sex, because of HRT. He could infect you. So anybody with whom you are not having regular sex should be asked to wear a condom; even though there is no risk of you becoming pregnant, he could give you vaginitis. The condom should be lubricated or your vagina may become sore.

Will my liver be damaged?

Hormones taken by mouth are absorbed from the intestines and pass through the liver where they very rarely, if ever, cause any damage unless it is already at risk because of previous attacks of jaundice. Hormones contained in patches and implants do not go through the liver like oral HRT and therefore do not affect it.

What will happen to my hair?

It should grow somewhat more luxuriantly. If, as rarely happens, the hair becomes thinner you may need to see a specialist in hair care (a trichologist).

What will happen to my skin?

In most cases it will look better and any elasticity which may be lost will return to it. Very, very few women on HRT develop acne and these have to alter the dose of HRT.

Is HRT likely to give me a heart condition?

Definitely not. Men are much more likely to die of heart disease than women of the same age, but post-menopausal women who do not take HRT have the same rates of heart attacks as men. It is virtually certain that the oestrogen part of hormone replacement treatment reduces the risk of coronary heart disease and of strokes. Women on HRT have as low a chance of having a heart attack as pre-menopausal women. Post-menopausal women who do not take HRT have much increased risks of heart attacks. HRT has been proved to lower the risks of heart attacks and possibly also of strokes to those of pre-menopausal women.

Can I drink alcohol while I am on HRT?

Definitely. It has been shown that up to two glasses of wine a day, especially red wine helps to protect against heart disease, as well as improving the quality of life. Excess drinking, particularly if you are already over-weight, can be dangerous for anyone taking or not taking HRT.

4

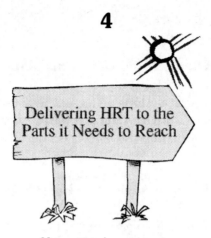

Delivering HRT to the Parts it Needs to Reach

Unopposed oestrogens
Combined oestrogen and progestogen tablets
Patches - Jellies or gels - Implants
The three monthly period tablets

You have decided with your family doctor or a spe-cialist at the menopause clinic to discuss which form of HRT you will take. The first question you may be asked is whether you have symptoms that need HRT or whether you want it to avoid trouble later. You will find that there is a bewildering choice of preparations, only one of which you can choose to take to start off with. But you are certainly not committed to your first choice if you do not like it when you start it; and anyhow it is probably a good idea to change the preparations from time to time until you find one that suits you so perfectly that you do not wish to stop it. If you are on the oral contraceptive pill and it suits you, you do not need to stop it, because the pill contains the hormones in HRT in still larger doses and can be taken for about two to three years after the menopause.

The box below points out the different groups of preparation on the market.

— Preparations available in the summer of 1996 —

✿ Unopposed oestrogen (for women who have had a hysterectomy)
✿ Tablets - seven different makes, all similar
✿ Patches - five different makes, all similar
✿ Skin gel - one preparation
✿ Local vaginal creams - four different makes
✿ Vaginal pessaries and tablets - three different makes
✿ Vaginal ring - one make (Estring)
✿ Combined oestrogen and progestogen tablets - 15 different strengths
✿ Patches and tablets - four different makes
✿ A combined hormone tablet causing little bleeding (Livial)

You may think that it is almost like choosing a car but if you are properly guided the choice is not nearly so difficult and for once the price hardly comes in to it. I say hardly because some packets of hormones contain two different preparations and there may be two prescription charges. It is also difficult to get an implant on the NHS and it may be quite expensive to have it privately.

If you are under private medical insurance or you are one of these who is just a private patient the price does enter in to it and perhaps you should enquire what it will cost.

Now to explain the different preparations in the box above.

'Unopposed' oestrogens
(for women who have had a hysterectomy)

The use of the word 'unopposed' may seem strange

but it is used because the ill effects of oestrogens on the lining of the womb (heaping up of the lining leading to heavy bleeding and worse), can be 'opposed' or countered by giving progesterone or substances like progesterone called progestogens. These preparations allow the uterus to bleed and the lining of the womb to be shed regularly so that it will not develop into a cancer at the worst.

Every woman who has not had a hysterectomy and is receiving oestrogens whether by tablet, patch, injection, ointment, or implant, has to take progestogens each month or at least every third month in order to have a period regularly and to cause the lining of the womb to shed and so avoid the risk of cancer developing there. So unopposed oestrogens are good for women who do not have a womb and therefore cannot develop cancer in it. And all others, even if they have reached their seventies, should take combined preparations and have a bleed, if not monthly at least once every three months. A comparatively new combined preparation (Livial) is said to cause very little bleeding unless it is taken within a year of the menopause. It should be reserved for women who are long past the menopause.

Why are there so many choices of oestrogens?

Because there are many different kinds of synthetic oestrogens. The one that is most usually used in a tablet is oestradiol, one of several factions also found in 'natural' preparations. Premarin contains natural oestrogens. It is prepared from pregnant mares' urine and contains at least four different kinds of oestrogen, whereas most of the synthetic ones contain just oestradiol.

The manufacturers - Wyeth - explained to me how they make Premarin which is the most widely prescribed of the natural oral oestrogens, in these words:

'The main active component of Premarin is a mixture of animal oestrogens which are extracted and purified from the urine of pregnant mares. The horses from which the oestrogens are obtained are located in Canada and the United States and are fed on a diet completely consisting of grains.

The horses are extremely well looked after according to high and established standards of care. Only the urine is used to produce the oestrogens and this is done without mistreating the horses in any way.

The oestrogens are extracted from the urine and subjected to a large number of purification steps before incorporation into tablets. The tablets are made by a conventional tabletting procedure.'

Combined Oestrogen and Progestogen tablets

These combined preparations of which there are 15 (in May 1996) contain oestrogen taken for the whole 25 days, opposed or countered by the progesterone-like tablets given for 12 days in the second half of the cycle. A few tablets (three different kinds) give the oestrogen and the progesterone in one tablet. Anyhow, at the end of 28 days bleeding should occur and the lining of the uterus be shed.

One of the commonly prescribed preparations is Prempak-C which is a pack of 28 maroon (or yellow double dose) tablets; containing the conjugated 'naturally' occurring oestrogens (Premarin) and 12 tablets of

Norgestrel which is a progestogen. So, the maroon or yellow tablet which delivers oestrogens is taken for all of the 28 days and the Progestogen for just the last 12 days of the cycle.

Usually a woman goes on immediately with a new pack after she has finished an old one without any interval of time. The stronger, yellow tablets are for those women who do not obtain adequate relief of their symptoms from the more commonly prescribed low dose oestrogens. Wyeth makes another similar preparation with a different progestogen (Premique).

Patches

Tablets that are swallowed are absorbed from the stomach and intestines into the blood stream and go through the liver before they are distributed around the body. The ways of avoiding this route into the general blood stream is by using patches or implants. Patches are applied to the skin through which the hormones are absorbed fairly slowly into the blood. Implants which are placed under the skin contain the hormones in small pellets which are absorbed very slowly over a period of six months or so.

Patches come in different strengths. They are applied to an area of skin which should be clean, dry and intact, which means not scratched or the site of a rash. They should not be applied near the breasts; so they are usually placed below the waistline; I recommend women to place them on their buttocks or the tops of the insides of their thighs in such a position that they would be hidden by a bikini. There is no need to advertise to all and sundry that you are taking oestrogens this way. In 1996 transparent patches came on the market and were less obvious than the older ones. The patches have only oestrogens in them and as they have not yet made a patch containing a progestogen as well, you have to take progestogen tablets for 12 days each month to make your womb bleed. There are three different makes. The patches are put on at about 3 - 4 day intervals so that you wear two fresh new patches a week, or eight a month. When you change over it is best to put the new patch in a slightly different place than the old one. One of the snags of these patches is that some women may be sensitive and come out in a localised rash but the transparent ones are less likely to cause this. The transparent ones suit all skin colours. They come in different doses. The oestrogen is contained in a fine mesh. Evorel made by Janssen-Cilag comes with four different strengths of oestrogen. Remember again that women who are wearing patches who still have a uterus have to take the Progestogen to have a bleed.

Jellies or Gels

In 1995 an ointment was put on the market in England for the first time, although it had been available in France for a few years beforehand, so it was well tried out. Oestrogel is a gel containing oestradiol. It is recommended that two measures of the gel be placed once a day on to the arms, shoulders or inner thighs. If the effect is not strong enough up to four measures a day can be used. As before, since oestrogel has to be opposed by women who still have a womb, it is important to take a progestogen tablet twelve days each cycle, unless you have had a hysterectomy.

Implants

Hormone implants are particularly successful for women who had a hysterectomy and who do not want to take tablets, put on patches, or use ointment. Usually two different hormones are inserted under the skin, one being a pellet containing oestradiol and another a pellet containing testosterone. The testosterone which is a male hormone has a wonderful effect on women who have lost their desire for sex - their libido. Many women who have had a hysterectomy find they have gone off sex, particularly if the ovaries have been removed at the same time as the womb. But even if they have not been removed, very often their blood supply is damaged and they do not produce enough of the right hormones. So an implant of the two pellets of oestradiol and testosterone seem to work magic in stopping hot flushes, irritability, insomnia and depression, but above all in improving libido in women who have had a hysterectomy. One patient put it *'I am fine now, but my poor husband can't keep up with me, whereas before I had to tell him I had a headache'*.

Testosterone makes women 'feel good' and look good too.

A few words of warning about implants. They should not be given to women who still have a uterus unless they are also prepared to take the progestogen tablets and they should not be repeated at intervals of less than 6 months. The effect is terrific for the first few months and then it gradually wears off, so that women come back demanding renewal of the implant in less than six months, but good doctors are not tempted to repeat the implant more than twice a year, because otherwise they would find the intervals getting shorter and shorter between each implant. Besides which, they are rather expensive; and they do involve making a cut in the skin, usually in the lower abdomen, so that they can be placed in the fat under the skin. The cut is made under a local anaesthetic. It is usually not necessary to put in a stitch. Pulling the edges of the cut together with a few strips of a narrow tape, Steri-Strip, will usually do the trick just as well. Very rarely a stitch may need inserting.

There are some women who do not like the idea of having a cut made for an implant to be inserted but still want the effect of testosterone. Although it is not often recommended some of these women can benefit from an injection of Sustanon. A small dose of this injection deeply placed into a muscle gives a depot that will last for several months and may be almost as effective as testosterone. It is not so highly recommended because unlike the implant which is absorbed very slowly over a period of six months, the Sustanon is absorbed more quickly. It has small risks of masculinising effects. These can be disturbing, as the voice may deepen and some hairs grow on the face. Only really experienced doctors should inject Sustanon and only small doses should be used. Regular visits to the doctor to see that no side effects are occurring should be made. Like the testosterone implant, Sustanon should not be repeated more than every 6 months or so. In any case only a small part of the lowest dose of Sustanon Depot can be used. Sustanon was developed for men who are deficient in the androgens they need for a full sex life, or to help them avoid or treat osteoporosis.

It was *not* developed for women to take. In the past there used to be small dose Testosterone tablets but these no longer seem to be made for sale in the UK; although they are becoming available in the United States in tablets containing oestrogens and small quantities of Testosterone (these are not yet licensed for sale in the UK).

Vaginal Creams

It seems logical for women whose main menopausal complaint is dryness in the vagina and maybe tightness there, to be given oestrogen at the place which is most deprived of it. Vaginal oestrogen creams have been invented just for that. They are pretty effective but rather messy. There are four different creams on the market to be placed in to the vagina with an applicator. The manufacturers say that one or two applicators full should be introduced in to the vagina daily for one or two weeks and after that only a half applicator full should be used. But, again because this is unopposed oestrogen the course should not last too long or if it does last for more than a month or two progestogen tables may need to be given. Also do not fill your vagina with oestrogen cream just before intercourse because you do not want your partner to be given oestrogens! Then it is better to use a lubricating jelly such as KY Jelly or Replens. Neither KY Jelly nor Replens contain any hormones at all. Or better still use a vaginal ring (see below).

There are also tablets that can be placed with an applicator in to the vagina, one daily for two weeks and then twice a week. Again, not too many nor too often because they are unopposed oestrogens.

Vaginal Rings (Estring) (Oestrogen ring)

A fairly recently marketed way of getting oestrogens to the vagina where it is most needed is in a plastic ring that is inserted high up into the vagina and worn continuously for three months. The ring should be replaced every three months and at present the recommendations are that it should not be used continuously for more than two years before 'giving it a rest'. The ring can be taken out by the woman herself before intercourse if it is in the way or she is worried that her partner might get a small 'dose' of oestrogen. The ring is of a standard size suitable for all women pushed high up into the vagina and delivers such small doses of oestrogens that it is very unlikely indeed to cause any changes in the uterus or in the breasts. It is used entirely for the treatment of dry vagina, painful intercourse and minor bladder disturbances such as the inability to hold urine properly. Patients much prefer it to oestrogen creams.

It may be important too to take Progestogen tablets to try to have a bleed every month or so, although the dose of oestrogens is so low that this bleeding may not occur.

The three monthly period tablets

Women who object to having monthly periods but would not mind having one every three months are now catered for with a preparation called Tridestra. The packs are made up of 91 tablets. Seventy of them contain Oestradiol of one kind and 14 contain a Progestogen together with the Oestrogen. There is an inactive preparation in the last seven tablets of the pack during which time the woman may well start a 'period'. Four bleeds a year (one every three months is almost certainly sufficient to protect the lining of the uterus from becoming cancerous while the dose of oestrogens is enough to prevent osteoporosis after the menopause.

5

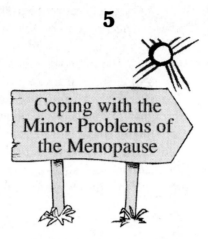

Coping with the
Minor Problems of
the Menopause

*Irritability - Lethargy - Depression
Coping with hot flushes
Unexpected periods*

All authorities and most books about the menopause
agree that *irritability* is the commonest of the minor
problems of the menopause. It may not appear so minor
when it irritates not only the woman but those around her
and it is certainly not such a minor problem if it leads to
conflict between your partner and yourself. If both of you
know that being irritable which is also defined as being
easily annoyed and peevish is more common at the time
of the menopause, that is half way to dealing with it. Most
people become irritable if they are irritated enough by
other people's behaviour, but when you become irritated
with yourself it may be wise to ask yourself why you have
become irritated. I think in many cases it is due to two
other common minor problems of the menopause, namely
forgetfulness and *lethargy*.

Forgetfulness in itself can be furiously annoying. It may be no comfort for the menopausal woman to realise that it is just one of the processes of ageing. If you had a wonderful memory all your life you are not likely suddenly to become a forgetful person, but if you, like most other people, tend to forget either to go to appointments or to find things that you have put down, and swear that it was in such and such a place when really you should have thought that it was in another place, you can take very minor measures to overcome this. Make notes and try not to forget where you have put them!

Irritability

Irritability, which is the commonest change in behaviour of the menopause requires that you are aware of being more irritable than you used to be and say to yourself after an outburst 'Why, oh why, oh why?' It is not easy to answer this question, but it is not sufficient to recognise this and expect other people to put up with it. I imagine that quite a lot of marital separation, even divorce comes about because of irritability and a little irrationality.

HRT is certainly a powerful weapon to combat this but irritability alone is not a good enough indication for starting on HRT. The best thing is to have a tolerant family and to be aware of the effect your irritability may have on those with whom you come in daily contact. There are no magic drugs for this.

Lethargy

Lethargy is an abnormal lack of energy. This may occur simply because of the menopause, but it may equally be because of overwork or some other form of illness or because of depression. I do not think that lethargy should just be accepted by a woman because she is menopausal. First of all she should check to see whether she really is lethargic. Can she get through as big a timetable of work and activity as ten years previously? Not many people can when they reach the age of say 60; but it should not be that difficult at the age of 50. One should have as much energy then, or nearly as much as 10 years previously. Lethargy may itself be due to anaemia and anaemia in its turn be due to abnormal vaginal bleeding. This is such an important accompaniment of the menopause for some women that there is a separate section on it (see page 64).

One patient came complaining of the most severe lethargy. This was at the time of her menopause, but seemed more extreme than one would have expected. The answer was revealed suddenly and rather unexpectedly when she was awoken in the middle of the night with most excruciating toothache. She went urgently to see her dentist. He took an x-ray which showed that she had an abscess round the root of a tooth. Almost miraculously when this was drained the pain immediately went (as expected) but also her energy seemed to come back within a day or two.

Bodily ills tend to become more frequent in the second half of one's life whether one is a man or a woman, and even before going to the doctor to have a 'check-up' the woman herself can think of things from the top of her head to the bottom of her feet which may be wrong. Tooth trouble is a common one. Many patients I have seen have calmly accepted they have a chronic cough. Only when they become lethargic they realise that the cough may be due to something more serious. It may not just be a smoker's cough. It may be due to some disease in the lungs and by this I do not only mean cancer, but chronic bronchitis and other lung diseases which especially affect people who have smoked fairly heavily all their lives. Such illnesses lead to lethargy.

Depression

A disgustingly large number of prescriptions are doled out by doctors and dispensed by chemists as anti-depressant drugs. They certainly do have a place in the treatment of depression but they act by-and-large more effectively after the menopause when combined with HRT. Depression can be serious in that it not only causes a most unpleasant series of mental states of hopelessness but also lessens the capacity to work effectively and to enjoy life. The one piece of advice which is rightly resented by people suffering from depression is 'pull yourself together'. This is just not possible. There is nothing to pull - no strings to tighten. Most women and men have phases when they are depressed and these usually pass but aid quite often needs to be given. It may just be a talk with a good friend or with a doctor. Sometimes help is needed from a counsellor. If depression gets more serious of course medical help may need to include the opinion 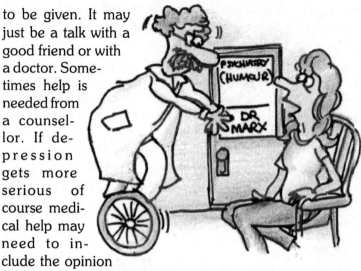 of a psychiatrist. There is no shame in seeking psychiatric help; often it is wonderfully effective. I work closely with a psychiatrist who if after talking to a patient thinks she requires medication usually works out with me what doses of hormones to give her together with the anti-depressant drugs.

A case study of a combination of symptoms

Here is the case of Mrs X who had an unpleasant combination of symptoms that were not very grave but still were serious enough to upset her life. She went through a very difficult menopause. Her story is told because it describes a combination of symptoms any of which commonly can occur without any serious permanent effects or damage. She had the lot.

Mrs X had to have her womb removed because it contained very large fibroids. They were not malignant but they kept on growing and her periods were becoming heavier and heavier. It took a lot of persuading her to have the operation which was absolutely essential for her health because she was becoming very anaemic, and the doses of iron her doctor was giving her were not sufficient to make up for her blood loss. Furthermore, her friends were noticing her abdomen swelling and asking her whether she was pregnant, which she was not. She would have loved to have had one more child but she did not become pregnant; and anyhow she was in her late forties and the fibroids in her uterus really ruled out pregnancy.

In removing the womb the surgeon could not avoid taking out one of her ovaries, but he hoped that the remaining ovary would be able to carry her through without a very sudden menopause occurring. Unfortunately the remaining ovary did not seem to contain any eggs at all, and the surgeon, when he was asked about it, was not at all certain that it would function to produce adequate amounts of hormones for her. It didn't. She refused HRT because she had heard 'such terrible things about it'.

Very soon after the operation she started to have symptoms of the menopause; the first and most depressing of which were severe night sweats. She woke up at night drenched in sweat, and had to change her nightdress once, twice or three times some nights. Although she slept in a double bed with her husband the bed covers on her side had to be removed or folded back so she risked and in fact sometimes caught cold. Nevertheless, she went on refusing hormone treatment although her surgeon wanted to give it to her. Her GP, who was most sympathetic, tried various sedatives but they only made her more depressed.

It was recognised that part of her depression was due to what is called 'the empty nursery syndrome'. She had children and got on extremely well with them, but as children do, they left home when they reached the right age. They did not have children themselves, so she had no grandchildren on whom she could pour out the great mother love that she had. She became very depressed indeed. Her general practitioner gave her stronger antidepressants. These hardly worked. She had always enjoyed sex with her husband, but her vagina had now become rather dry and that put him off somewhat; as did the fact that she sweated so much at night. They were still however, very much in love with one another. She then developed *hot flushes during the day*, and felt that she could not go on coping with her social life.

The firm for which she worked was sold and she was made redundant - bad for her morale. Eventually in despair her general practitioner sent her back to the surgeon who was finally able to persuade her to have HRT.

He chose implants for three reasons. The first was to make sure that she had HRT which would last at least six months. She could not stop the course at a whim because the hormones were implanted into her. The second reason was to give her plenty of oestrogen and the third to give her testosterone to help her with her libido and to want her husband again.

The effect was almost dramatic. Within a week or so of the implant the night sweats stopped and within two or three months her vagina felt good to her and welcoming to her husband.

But she still had nagging fears about the possibility of developing cancer of the breast and these fears were not made any less because her breasts did become a little tender as they often do with HRT. A mammogram reassured her. She agreed to have another implant six months after the first one and she had four more in the following three years.

Then she asked to be given a trial without them. She had long come off the antidepressants, and in fact she had not needed them at all a month or two after starting her HRT (though sometimes the effect of HRT may take four months to be felt fully).

To her happy surprise once the implants were stopped the night sweats which she had feared would come back *did not* return. Nor did the depression. Later, her husband in his turn became redundant; but they now had two pensions and they were able to cope well financially. The hobbies they developed together have drawn them closer and closer. Love of music, dancing, and long walks in the country are not only good occupations for them to undertake together, but healthy exercise for both of them, which is most essential to help avoid the development of osteoporosis.

This is a success story of a severe menopause; fortunately highly successfully treated with, initially, antidepressant drugs (in her case fairly useless) and oestrogens and testosterone. She regularly still attends for follow-ups to make quite sure that her breasts are quite safe. She has a mammogram every three years. Her breasts are now firm but not at all tender; and her vagina is moist and supple thanks to the hormones she had for three years and thanks to regular sexual intercourse.

Incidentally, I mentioned that Mrs X suffered from the *empty nest syndrome*. Not all menopausal women have empty nests. One woman started her second family on re-marrying at the age of 44. Soon after she found herself going through the menopause when her new baby was still a small toddler. This can and increasingly may happen to women who have put off having babies until well established in their careers or who have remarried after divorce. One woman said to me, 'We have five children - two of his, two of mine, and one of ours, and now the menopause!'

Coping with hot flushes

For about three quarters of all women at some time during the menopause, hot flushes are at the least a slight nuisance and at the worst an acute embarrassment. Sometimes women when they first experience hot flushing think this is just like the blushing that occurred when they were young and going through puberty. But of course it is not the same. An emotional blush which can still happen at any stage of life for men as well as women affects different parts from the menopausal blush. At the menopause there is an increased flow of blood through the hands and forearms. The emotional blush is almost entirely felt in the face. The blush in the menopause is entirely in the skin, mainly in the face, the hands and the chest, but not in the muscles. The flushes very seldom last for more than six minutes at the most but usually less. It is very difficult to explain why some women have these flushes for years whereas others are over them within a few months.

Here are some very sensible suggestions that have been made to me by patients:

✿ If you are going to work and your work involves going into other people's offices a lot, do dress in such a way that you can shed layers of clothing if you feel hot and put them on again after the flush has stopped or before going out into the street. It is good to stop wearing anything made of wool and of velvet; instead wear three and sometimes even four layers of light fabrics. The one nearest the body should always be sleeveless and might well be covered by another sleeveless garment. On top of that you could wear a light jacket or pullovers which can be shed and put on again

✿ Some offices are quite unexpectedly warm and so shedding a layer or two unobtrusively is sensible. But, do put them on again before going in to cooler surroundings. Each morning when dressing to go out do work out a strategy for coping if you are going to be unexpectedly overtaken by a hot flush in the place you are visiting

✿ The menopause, which is a wonderful time for being more active and for travelling and for entertaining and being entertained, is also a time for a lot of women to acquire a new wardrobe. This should be designed so that layers can be put on and taken off. It is a good idea in the morning to calculate where you are likely to be and what to put on so that you will still be smart no matter how many layers of light clothing you are wearing

✿ One patient of mine in the summer months when it would not appear too obvious would walk around with a hand-held battery fan which she switched on as soon as she felt a hot flush coming on her face.

✿ One article of clothing that is a particular nuisance to women who have hot flushes is tights. Furthermore tights worn over synthetic material panties do not allow sweat to disperse easily and if you have once had an attack of Thrush it is quite likely to recur

✿ Here is a useful tip from a patient. She always travels with a little anti-fungal ointment such as Gynodaktrin in her wash bag. If she had a bleed or even if she did not, when she thought she was going to develop an attack of thrush she would put a dab or two of the Gynodaktarin cream on a tampon and insert it. The manufacturers do make tampons which have Gynodaktarin incorporated, but this 'home made' product seems a sensible one and may be cheaper

Unexpected periods

Periods often do not stop suddenly but become spaced out and one may appear quite unexpectedly. Women who have a very active life are used to thinking positively and this is a good time to do so. The menopause is the first time for many women for thirty years or so not to have to worry about periods or what to take away in sanitary protection just in case a period is due. Most women however can tell when a period is likely to come on because of an extra firmness of the breasts and a little heaviness in the days before bleeding may be expected. If this is the case, it may be necessary to wear a thick pantyliner for a few days.

Migraine

Whereas headache can occur quite often at the menopause, migraine from which a woman may have suffered for years, tends to stop. Migraine is a rather special kind of headache. It is more common in women than in men. It comes at intervals and lasts anything from 2 to 72 hours. There is no headache between the attacks and all attacks start with some changes in vision such as a kind of aura or a sensitivity to light during the attacks. Quite often there are also changes in the intestine. Migraine can occur in girls as young as seven, but more often at puberty and later. Some women get it before their periods and some when they start the contraceptive pill, but other women are relieved of their migraine headaches while taking the pill. Pregnant women very rarely have migraine attacks but the attacks do tend to return after the baby is born. Migraine seems to be due to hormones circulating in the brain and as the hormone levels drop off at the menopause, migraine does too. 'Ordinary' headaches can become more frequent at the menopause, but they may be due to worries or to insomnia which itself affects nearly half of all women at the menopause. In some this too does not tend to last for long.

Giddiness

Some women after the menopause complain of attacks of giddiness. If your doctor can find no other reason for these 'giddy spells' then if you are not already taking HRT perhaps you can get him to prescribe some and in many cases you will be pleasantly surprised that these spells become far less frequent or even stop altogether.

Sex Life and the Menopause

Obviously by the time a woman reaches her late forties or early fifties she is less likely to be as sexually active as she was in her late teens or early twenties. Libido, which is the desire for sexual contact, often however, increases once some of the worries of the reproductive age have gone. Most women have an increase in libido at and soon after the menopause, and many find their sex lives better even without taking any HRT. This is because their adrenal glands go on manufacturing testosterone now the ovaries are manufacturing a little less oestrogen. It is testosterone that makes you feel 'raunchy'; and there is proportionately more of it.

Libido is partly due to the way your head and your heart as well as your hormones work. The head and the heart are more important than the hormones. If your heart is in the right place and you still love your partner very much but find you do not have strong sex feelings for him when he tries to arouse you, then hormones are the answer. These include oestrogens, and for some women testosterone - available in the UK at present only in implant form.

Lessening of libido

Only about 25% of all women find that their libido (desire for sexual activity) goes down at the menopause. One of the commonest reasons for this is that intercourse may become painful if the vagina has become dry because of lack of oestrogens. There can be an annoying combination of an increased desire for sexual activity because the adrenal glands are making relatively more testosterone and the ovaries are making less oestrogen. This means that though the wish is there the performance becomes painful. That inevitably puts both of the couple off. The increased proportion of testosterone makes you feel 'raunchy' but the soreness in the vagina takes much of the pleasure away. Things to avoid if the vagina becomes tight or too sore are douches which wash away the natural contents of the vagina and leave it thinner and less elastic.

Talc powders, perfumes and perfumed soap should not be put on the labia because the skin becomes very dry and it may be necessary to counter this dryness with skin softening creams. The vagina should be moist and slippery and a preparation called 'Replens' has been developed in order to help the vagina stay moist. There are slight disadvantages in this in that it cannot be prescribed on the National Health Service and it is very expensive in that a month's supply costs £13.00. It does seem that the newly developed Estring is a cheaper and more effective way of countering vaginal dryness (see page 46).

Bladder control and the menopause

It is not generally realised how many women from their school days on- wards, find it a little difficult to avoid passing a few drops of urine, 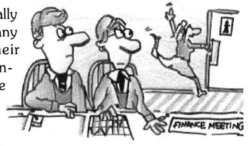 particularly when performing various strenuous exercises. Girls do not often complain to other people about it, but just wear pantyliners to absorb any drops of urine they pass involuntarily. Because they do not com- plain people are not aware of how common this minor incontinence is. Involuntary loss of urine tends to become more frequent at and after the menopause. This is due to some loss of collagen which gives elasticity to the tissues in the pelvis. The vagina, the bladder and the pipe from the bladder to the outside (the urethra) sometimes lose some of their elasticity and flexibility. HRT and particularly the newest forms of HRT such as the Estring vaginal pessary containing oestrogen are very helpful in combating this nuisance.

Many hospitals and some general practices that have menopause clinics have a physiotherapist working in them who specialises in teaching bladder control methods to women with involuntary loss of urine, which is sometimes due to prolapse and is much more common in the menopause because of the loss of elasticity.

There are many operations that have been designed for incontinence with or without prolapse and if it is seriously worrying then it is important to seek help and possibly surgery for this very embarrassing condition which may make a normal social life very difficult.

6

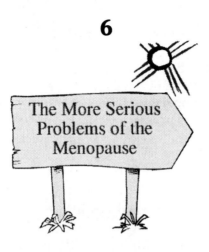

The More Serious
Problems of the
Menopause

Unusual vaginal bleeding
Hysteroscopy
Endometrial resection
Hysterectomy

It is not surprising that the pattern of bleeding as the menopause approaches should change. This is due in nearly all cases to the lessening of oestrogen and of progesterone production by the ovaries. Production of both these hormones will diminish when there are no eggs left to be released. The feedback to the pituitary gland which has been explained may occur somewhat differently for oestrogens and progestogens. In consequence FSH and LH production may occur differently with alterations in the periods. Most often the periods just diminish and sometimes stop but occasionally they may be heavier for a short time. This does not matter providing that it is for a short time and providing that the periods are not very heavy. It certainly does not matter at all if the periods are becoming lighter and more spaced out, because that is quite normal and to be expected.

There are other glands in the body that make hormones and particularly the adrenal glands that make some testosterone helping the woman to have a good libido and also helping the periods not to be too heavy. Heavy periods can be a nuisance and more than a nuisance if they lead to anaemia.

Heavy periods

There are many things that doctors can do when patients complain of heavy periods. The first and most important one is to examine the uterus very carefully in order to ascertain whether it is larger than normal and in particularly whether there are any fibroids in it, because fibroids may be the cause of heavy periods. Nobody knows for certain why fibroids which are non-malignant lumps in the uterus develop.

At the same time as the doctor examines the uterus he also feels for cysts in the ovaries; and if a smear test has not been taken during the previous year he should take a smear. This is now a routine, for which general practitioners are paid by the NHS. A smear is taken with the newest kind of spatula which picks up cells not only from the neck of the womb but also from inside the lining of the neck of the womb and if there are any seriously abnormal cells in the lower part of the body of the uterus they are picked up also. The smears the doctor or nurse takes have to be sent to the laboratory to be read.

A scan is arranged if the uterus appears to be bigger than normal. This scan gives the doctor accurate measurements about the size of the uterus and also tells him about the state of the ovaries. Furthermore it shows him where any fibroids or other abnormalities in the uterus are situated.

Once the initial tests have shown that there is no evidence of any cancer or precancerous condition (from the smears) and the uterus is a normal size, the doctor may make correctly a diagnosis of 'dysfunctional bleeding'. This simply means that the action of the hormones is not as well balanced as it should be.

Dysfunctional bleeding - Non-hormone treatments

There are two ways of tackling this kind of bleeding if it is heavy. The first is to use a preparation that is not made of hormones but acts on the blood vessels in the uterus. There are three very good ones on the market called Dicynene (Ethamsylate), Cyklokapron (Tranexamic Acid) as well as Ponstan (Mefenamic Acid). None of these three preparations contain any hormones and all are very safe. Although every single drug that anyone can take can have side effects, they are very rare with these three drugs. Incidentally, a simple drug such as aspirin can have side effects such as making abnormal bleeding from the uterus much heavier, so taking aspirin is not a good idea if you are having heavy, painful periods.

Hormone preparations for dysfunctional bleeding

There are several oral hormone preparations which raise the level of progestogen to lessen the amount of blood that is lost. These are Duphaston, Gestone, Provera and others. Danol is another hormone preparation taken by mouth.

There are still others given as a depot in muscles that speed up the process of the menopause by acting like the hypothalamus does when it shuts off production of FSH and LH. This depot is a releasing hormone analogue, which means that it works like the releasing hormones sent out by the hypothalmus. This last kind of preparation thins the lining of the womb very quickly. It can also lessen the size of fibroids and is particularly useful before operations if they are going to be difficult to remove. This is helpful to the surgeon if a woman just wants her fibroids removed (but not her uterus taken out) as she will do if she still wants to retain the possibility of having children after the fibroids have been removed.

When the heavy bleeding has led to anaemia iron preparations are usually given in tablet form, or sometimes in linctuses to drink.

If none of these measures is appropriate or fail to work gynaecologists resort to surgery. What they do and how they do it really depends on what they have found in their examination of the patient. The ultrasound scans have told them about the size of the uterus and its shape, whether there are fibroids present and where in the uterus they are, and whether there are cysts in an ovary.

But above all, the gynaecologist can see how thick the lining of the womb is. With a thin lining before a period is due it is not likely to be heavy, but with a thick one it is very likely to be so.

New procedures

Hysteroscopy

A new procedure is becoming popular in gynaecological out patients departments. It does not require an anaesthetic, although it can be slightly uncomfortable. It is called hysteroscopy. In this procedure the doctor inserts a small telescope into the uterus with which he can see the lining of the uterus very accurately. Using it he can also remove polyps, which are a frequent cause of heavy bleeding, especially around the menopause. Sometimes hysteroscopy and the procedures that are carried out through the hysteroscope are all that is needed.

Until recently the operation of dilatation and curettage was carried out extensively, but hysteroscopy allows for a more accurate evaluation of the state of the lining of the womb and in many cases has done away with the need for dilatation and curettage as a method of diagnosis. Gynaecologists still, however, carry out dilatation and curettage to scrape away most of the lining of the womb, hoping that this will be effective in reducing the blood loss until the menopause takes over. Furthermore, the scrapings are sent to the laboratory for an accurate diagnosis to be made of the state of the lining of the uterus.

Endometrial resection

Until recently hysterectomy was the standby to remove the womb, and of course, with it its lining. All gone forever. But, within the last ten years or so, a new procedure, *endometrial resection*, has become popular. Endometrial resection means more than dilatation and curettage because the lining of the womb is not only scraped out but burnt out with a curette delivering diathermy, or a small ball delivering diathermy, or the lining is removed by using laser through the hysteroscope. It was greeted with enthusiasm by large groups of gynaecologists, but the follow-up results three or four years after the operation have shown that women are less satisfied with it than they are with hysterectomy. They are less satisfied because bleeding quite often does not stop completely while the symptoms of pre-menstrual tension and other annoyances still persist, as does a small risk of pregnancy and therefore a need for contraception.

Hysterectomy

Hysterectomy is still the ultimate treatment for women with heavy periods who no longer wish to have children and who want to get back to work and regain their fitness.

One patient is the administrator of a large charity. Her heavy periods were 'really getting her down'. She was well informed of all the choices available to her, and she elected to have a hysterectomy. She is a 'no messing-about lady' who found out which ways hysterectomy can be performed. These are:

✿ Through a cut in the abdomen, called a 'bikini' cut which allows the gynaecologist to remove the uterus and if he wishes the cervix and the ovaries, through a cut, the scar of which can be completely hidden under even a small bikini Dr John Studd, who is a great advocate of HRT, thinks all women over the age of 45 should have their ovaries removed at the same time as hysterectomy and should be given an implant of HRT during the operation. Other gynaecologists think that the hormonal changes of the menopause should be allowed to come about naturally, even if the woman does not have a uterus but with the ovaries left behind

✿ The second way of removing the uterus is vaginally. This operation is ideal if the uterus is not very large and can be moved around fairly easily. It is a most effective and satisfactory operation and leaves no visible scar

✿ The third way is by laparoscopy assisted vaginal hysterectomy. This operation is particularly good to help to free the uterus from its attachments by looking through a laparoscope inserted through the navel in the abdomen and by cutting and tying of the blood vessels near the top of the uterus by techniques using the laparoscope. The surgeon then proceeds to remove the uterus through the vagina. It is relatively easy because the uterus has been freed from its upper supporting structures and can be brought out through the vagina much more easily in most cases. The advantage of this third procedure over abdominal hysterectomy is that there is much less pain. The healing process is much quicker, so that the woman, like the charity administrator lady can get back to work very quickly, say in two weeks, rather than two months which is the normal recovery period after an abdominal hysterectomy

What is certain, is once the uterus is out there can be no further chance of any pregnancy, no further vaginal bleeding, and no chance of cancer developing in it. In all these methods the top of the vagina is carefully sewn up so that the scar is there at the top of the vagina but with vaginal hysterectomy there is no visible scar at all because it is all hidden in the vagina. With laparoscopically assisted vaginal hysterectomy there are three small scars on the lower abdomen as compared with the one continuous scar well hidden by a bikini. Strangely enough, many women prefer to have a bikini cut than have three small scars, chiefly because of the position of the scars.

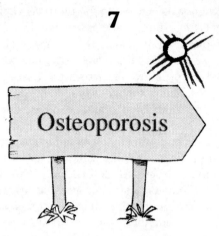

7

Osteoporosis

Who suffers from osteoporosis?
Bone density is all important
Non-hormonal treatment
Prevention of osteoporosis

In osteoporosis bones become weakened because of loss of some of their minerals. The total mass of bone becomes less than normal, and the tissue of the bone becomes fragile so that it is at risk of breaking. The bones become porous. It is a common, serious condition. If someone with osteoporosis falls on her wrist or hip it is more likely to fracture. While healthy bones have holes in them like a tight honeycomb, in osteoporosis the holes have become so big that the structure of the bone is much weakened.

Who suffers from osteoporosis?

Mainly women. But some children are born with

fragile bones. Girls who are anorexic tend to develop it because tissue is lost from the bones. Men also can have osteoporosis but women are four times more likely to develop it.

The bone weakening starts at about the age of 40 and becomes worse directly after the menopause. About 1% of the bone mass is lost every year. Men do not often develop osteoporosis before the age of 50 although there are quite a number of elderly men with hump backs due to osteoporosis. One sees them, but few realise why the former upright man becomes a little folded, and needs a stick to walk due to his osteoporosis.

Women develop it if they are deprived of female hormones at and after the menopause. Young girls who are anorexic develop it because of the absence of the correct minerals due to their not eating properly, and because of hormone disturbances which also lead them to not having periods.

About one quarter of all women at the age of about 70 have 'silent' small fractures in the front of the bones of their spine. This gives them the famous 'Dowager's hump' with loss of height as the vertebrae tend to fold up a little.

Small fractures of the vertebrae occur without symptoms, except for the loss of some height. These fractures lead to the excess forward curvature of the spine known technically as kyphosis (Humpback). More rarely there is some sideways curvature of the spine known as scoliosis.

After the menopause there is also some loss of collagen, which is a group of proteins that occurs in bones, cartilage and the deeper layers of the skin. The skin becomes thinner and tissues sag a little. There is quite often some loss of hair. The teeth may become loose because of weakening of the bones of the jaws. They may even fall out or have to be removed if there was some infection around the roots of the teeth or in the gums. HRT greatly lessens the likelihood of losing teeth after the menopause.

While a quarter of all women risk developing osteoporosis by the age of 60, half have it by the age of 70. One third of all hospital orthopaedic beds are taken up by patients as a result of their having osteoporosis. In the UK there are probably about 60,000 women who have had hip fractures, 50,000 who have had fractures of their wrists and 40,000 who have had small fractures of their spines, and incredibly another 50,000 who have had fractures of other bones. These are very large numbers and what a waste!

Because the spine fractures do not often give rise to pain, nine tenths of these are never diagnosed unless x-rays are taken.

The cost to the country is enormous. Fractured hips alone cost hospitals about £180 million a year. If a bone has become deformed no treatment, except occasionally an operation to correct the deformity is necessary, but if it has become fractured like in the hip then certainly an operation to fix it is necessary although it will not alter the deformity. Some of the newer medical treatments can alter the density of bone and bring it back to normal, so that while the deformity cannot be improved further progress is stopped.

Osteoporosis altogether costs this country about £750 million a year. Fracturing your hip if you are an old lady increases your chance of dying earlier, in part because you cannot look after yourself properly and partly because staying in bed gives rise to an increased likelihood of thrombosis, pneumonia and pressure sores as well as of bladder infection. Worst of all however, is, the dependence on help from others. Fractured arms are less upsetting than fractured hips, but can be painful and may require an anaesthetic to set them and need four to six weeks in plaster for them to heal.

Bone density is all important

How can we predict which women are most likely to be candidates for osteoporosis? By measuring the bone density. This means assessing the thickness of the bone due to its mineral content. From the time we are born until before puberty there is a gradual progressive increase in the density of bones. This is accelerated in the two or three years before and after puberty when girls tend to grow fairly rapidly. By puberty the bone has reached about 90% of its density, and this gradually increases to its full level by the age of about 40. Bone density can vary according to inheritance, and what a woman has done with her life. Women who are athletic, but not too athletic, develop denser bones than those who sit around. Heavy smoking and drinking excess alcohol (more than 3 units a day - one unit being the amount in a glass of wine) lessens bone density. Lying in bed immobilised because of illness makes bone density go down further. Space travellers it so happens, also lose bone density if they stay up in space for any length of time.

Women who have an early natural menopause or are menopausal because of operations or x-rays are prone to develop low density bone structure. Female athletes who over exercise may lose some of their bone density.

Measuring bone density
While the strength of bone cannot be measured it is

possible now to measure fairly accurately, the density of bones. The risk of later suffering a fracture can be worked out by readings obtained. A risk does not predict that a fracture *will* occur, only that it is more *likely* to occur. The risks are very low indeed for those with good thick bone structure, but increase as the bones thin. Diet plays an important part. If there is too little calcium and vitamin D in the food, bone density lessens. The density is measured by a special x-ray machine (called technically the dual x-ray absorptiometer, or for short DXA). Health authorities are responsible for seeing that densitometry machines exist in their areas. These deliver very low dosage x-rays so there is no need to worry about damage from the x-rays. There is not even any need to undress to have a densitometry examination as the x-rays can 'look through' most clothing and give the specialist who is used to reading these pictures a very accurate measurement of the density of the spinal bones which are those which are most commonly examined. It is possible to examine wrist bones. Although there are quite large numbers of special densitometry machines around the country they are not fully used, because there are not enough specialist radiographers available to make full use of them. It is a little bit like buying a very expensive car and taking it out only for a half day at weekends. Ordinary x-rays are really no good in diagnosing bone density.

The prevention of osteoporosis and fractures due to it

The main cause of osteoporosis in women is the gradual lessening of the amount of oestrogen circulating in the blood. Oestrogen prevents bone loss. HRT is not only good for many of the other symptoms of the menopause but also good for bones. The amount each woman takes should be worked out according to her needs and her body build. Apart from the giving of hormones there are other factors in the lifestyle before the menopause that are helpful to avoid bone density going down, and even increase bone density in those who have lost some bone structure.

Calcium is an important food, particularly in dairy products such as milk, butter and cheese. Vitamin D is necessary in the diet to help calcium being absorbed.

Calcium tablets are not very well absorbed and that is why they are so seldom prescribed. They only can help when combined with other treatments such as hormone therapy but there is now a new drug which is claimed partially to reverse osteoporosis. This drug is called Fosomax and will be discussed a little later in this chapter.

Non-hormonal treatment

Etidronate, a non-hormone treatment has been used for the past ten years or so. It is one of a group of chemicals called 'biphosphonates'. It is also called Didronel PMO. It is a phosphonate with added calcium, especially indicated if there is osteoporosis in the spine. One tablet of Didronel is taken daily for fourteen days; followed by one tablet containing calcium carbonate daily in water for 26 days. The packet contains full instructions on how the tablets should be taken in cycles of 92 days for up to three years. The diet should contain enough calcium and vitamin D. Didronel is usually only prescribed for women who are ten to fifteen years past the menopause and who have back pain and some loss of height. Didronel, which is not a hormone will not have any effect on hot flushes, sweats and so on. It does not prevent osteoporosis, and is usually prescribed only for those women who are not taking HRT. Doctors do not yet know whether adding Didronel to HRT is going to be helpful.

Fosamax is another phosphonate prescribed for osteoporosis after the menopause. It is taken daily in the morning with a full glass of water twenty minutes before food. It is still a fairly new drug and doctors, as with every new drug, are urged to watch carefully to see whether side effects develop. These seem to occur rarely but include pain in the abdomen and occasionally a rash. If this happens stop taking Fosamax.

Prevention of osteoporosis

Osteoporosis can be prevented by correct lifestyle, adequate diet and avoiding over indulgence of alcohol and taking sufficient, but not excessive exercise.

However, HRT is the most effective measure for preventing osteoporosis and for treating it once it has been diagnosed. It cannot be taken late to help with a bone that has already been fractured, but it may prevent new fractures occurring. Preferably it should be started at or very soon after the menopause and continued for several years under prescription from your doctor.

Where to go for help and obtain more information about osteoporosis

The National Osteoporosis Society disseminates information about osteoporosis and increases awareness of the condition. In this way it helps women avoid it, and to cope with it once it has occurred. The National Osteoporosis Society has some very eminent doctors on its committee.

This remarkable society is funded almost entirely by patients who have suffered or are suffering from osteoporosis and are being helped. It receives no government funding but works happily with the government and the National Health Service.

8

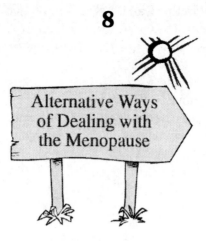

Self-help methods
Homeopathy treatment
Herbal remedies

At the start of this chapter I repeat that the menopause is not an illness, nor is it the cause of any other illnesses. It is just a period of time that marks the change from the reproductive years to the non-reproductive phase of life. Many women notice few, if any, of the long list of symptoms that have appeared in previous chapters.

Here are a few self-help methods to avoid some of the very minor symptoms.

Self help methods:
- ✪ Do not be embarrassed by your hot flushes. They are much more noticeable to you than the people around you
- ✪ Avoid rushing to get to places. That alone can make you flushed and it is better to plan your day well
- ✪ Wear layers of clothes rather than one or two heavy garments (explained on pages 56-57)

✪ Drink cold drinks because hot tea and coffee and spiced foods make hot flushes worse. Avoid them if you are out or drink them at home where you are not embarrassed by having a hot flush or two

✪ The bedroom should be cool. Rarely you and your partner may have to sleep in separate beds, but only for a short time

✪ Stop smoking

✪ Do have your doctor check your heart, your blood pressure, your breasts, your uterus, and do have cervical smears regularly if you still have your womb

✪ Do not stop contraceptive methods until you are at least a year past your last period

✪ Do not become an HRT addict. This means do not take extra doses of oestrogens in order to raise your levels of oestrogens. If you do then use something like oestrogel which you rub into the forearm. This is easy to use and can give you only small extra doses of hormones if you feel you need them

✪ Avoid going out in the sun. Women at the menopause tend to sunburn very easily because a lack of production of melanin, which is the pigment in the blood that allows you to go brown instead of red on exposure to sun. Sunbathing is far less fashionable now than it was a few years ago

✪ Menopause clinics are there to help you so use them

✪ Do not hesitate to use pain killers if you have headaches

✪ Do go to your doctor if you have changes in your bowel habits such as constipation, or particularly bleeding from the back passage. This has nothing to do with the menopause and does require attention from your doctor

✪ Add certain important oils to your diet, namely Oil of Evening Primrose and Fish Oils. Eat plenty of fish

✪ A proprietary preparation called Efacal containing Evening Primrose Oil, Fish Oil and calcium is a useful one on the market

Many women seek alternative methods other than

those already mentioned under 'self help' above, when dealing with the menopause. They do not like HRT and its side effects; and in truth side effects do arise from it in some women. No patient has all of them, but the list includes:

- ✪ breast tenderness
- ✪ occasional nausea
- ✪ occasional cramps in the legs
- ✪ weight gain
- ✪ headaches
- ✪ stomach discomfort
- ✪ bloating if too high a dose of progesterone is used
- ✪ irritability (although often improved and not made worse by HRT)
- ✪ various aches and pains

One of my patients refused HRT saying that she was frightened of all the above side-effects which she listed to me. She also, probably correctly, felt that the menopause was being over medicalised. She told me, sensibly in her case, that a natural phenomenon such as the menopause should not need medicines to enable a woman to go through with it, or to cope with the symptoms that she had which were quite real. In any case 50% of women on HRT give it up after about five years, mostly because of the annoyance of having to bleed every month, and also because of the fear, particularly of developing breast cancer (see page 27). My patient's main complaint was her rather severe hot flushes. Her answer was to take homoeopathic remedies.

She took *Lachesis* for her hot flushes, *Bryonia* for her vaginal dryness and *Folliculum* for the slightly irregular bleeding that she had just before her periods stopped. She took all these in homoeopathic doses. She claimed certainly to her own satisfaction, and I understand from her to the satisfaction of many other women, that these doses of these forms of homoeopathy are most effective. The remedies, the Lachesis and Folliculum were taken at 6c potency (the 'c' is an indication of the concentration of the drug in water).

A German homoeopathic medicine called Mulimen is specifically used for treating symptoms of the menopause.

Homoeopathy uses very small doses of drugs diluted many times. Homoeopathic drugs can be obtained from shops that specialise in them or from homoeopathic health centres.

Six different homoeopathic drugs are widely prescribed for the menopause. Homoeopathic practitioners emphasise that the taking of drugs must be tailored to the particular needs of each patient. It is really not good enough to go into a shop that sells homoeopathic drugs and order without consulting a special practitioner in this subject. Nevertheless, here's a list of homoeopathic drugs that I have been told (I do not practice homoeopathy myself) are worth taking:

✿ Ambra D4 20%
✿ Cimci Fuga Racemosa D6 25%
✿ Lachesis Muta D12 10%
✿ Sanguinaria c D12 10%
✿ Sepia D6 25%
✿ Zincum Metallicum DS 10%

All these preparation are in 50% alcohol and the D is the dilution. My patient is actually taking 15 - 20 drops of a mixed preparation of all these six drugs diluted in a small liqueur glass of ordinary tap water.

If you wish to know more about homoeopathic treatment of the menopause do read a very informative book published by Insight Publications and written by Dr Trevor Smith. It is entitled 'Homoeopathy for the Menopause'.

Herbal Remedies

Herbal remedies are not homoeopathic drugs. They are sold to be taken either as a herbal infusion (like tea) or as a tincture in alcohol. They are also dispensed as pills and can be obtained from shops that specialise in selling herbal medicines. Herbal medicines are not always without danger. The title herbal medicine may seem to indicate that the drugs are absolutely safe. This is not so, especially with Chinese herbal medicines. Some of them are very toxic and must be taken with great care and under medical advice. Nevertheless, here is a list of herbal medicines taken by some of my patients:

✿ Vltex Agnus Castur
✿ Black Coroosh
✿ Agnus castur is said to stimulate the production of progesterone and even may contain progesterone substances in it. Other infusions patients have taken with success are IK Donqui (tanqui) and Chamaelirium Luteum
✿ Vitamin A (but it must be taken in the correct doses because too high doses are dangerous), can help to combat thinning of bones
✿ Vitamin B, again if taken in the correct doses may help with vaginal dryness
✿ There are many vegetables that in themselves contain oestrogen-like substances. Particularly the seeds of flax and the cheese-like substance Tofu, which many Japanese women eat. It is a soft, fairly tasteless substance that looks like cheese and it does seem to contain natural oestrogens
✿ Mexican yam does contain oestrogen-like substances and commercial oestrogens are made from Mexican yam in many cases.

Yoga exercises may very well help at the menopause but start doing them very gently at first and do them under instruction from a fully qualified practitioner. One or two of my patients swear by them. One certainly stands on her head at least once a day. This is a perfectly rational measure for improving the circulation and for keeping young. Lord Yehudi Menuhin claims that 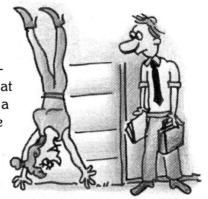 much of his great energy and enthusiasm for life is helped by practising Yoga for many years of his long life. It is becoming more popular as a form of treatment, and it is sensible when practised under the eye of a good teacher. It is certainly very safe.

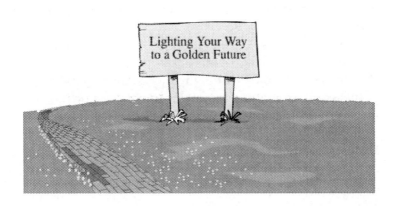

Lighting Your Way
to a Golden Future

9

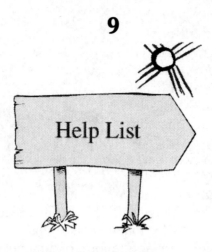

(i) Glossary

Artificial Menopause Brought about when the function of the ovaries is stopped by a doctor either removing them at an operation or giving radiotherapy or chemotherapy. The effects are the same as a natural menopause but are often sudden and more severe

Cervix Neck of the womb

Climacteric (from the Greek 'rung of a ladder') Another word for the menopause

Collagen Fibres, yellow strands of tissue which are packed close in the ligaments

Dilatation and curettage Involves stretching the neck of the womb so that a scraping instrument can be passed through it in order to scrape some of the lining of the womb away usually for examination in a laboratory

Dowagers hump Occurs because the front edges of some of the vertebrae in the upper chest and lower part of the neck weaken and collapse slightly, tilting the vertebral column forwards

Endometrium The lining of the womb. At puberty it thickens and is shed with the first period. After that it thickens in such a way as to be able to receive a fertilised egg. Each month if there is no egg to be implanted the endometrium is shed with the blood of the menstrual period. A thin layer of endometrium, however, is left for new endometrium to grow in the following month

Endometrial ablation Destruction of the lining of the womb by burning it with diathermy or with laser

The Feedback Mechanism Comes into play when the level of the hormone produced as a result of the action of a stimulating hormone rises so high that its excess in the blood stream 'feeds-back' to the organ making the stimulating hormone to tell it to slow down. So, a high level of oestrogen feeds-back to the pituitary gland to 'tell it' to slow down or stop FSH production. At the menopause there is insufficient oestrogen to feed-back to the pituitary gland so FSH production rises to very high levels

Follicle Stimulating Hormone (FSH) Made in the pituitary gland and acts mainly on the ovaries to ripen the follicles in which the eggs are stored and these ripe follicles produce oestrogens

Hormones Substances produced by glandular tissue in organs such as the thyroid gland, the ovaries, the adrenal glands etc. These substances are all released into the blood stream to reach those organs which are their targets

Hypothalamus Sometimes called the olive, because of its shape and size is situated in the base of the brain. It produces gonadotrophin releasing hormones (GnRH) which trigger the pituitary gland to make follicle stimulating hormone at the correct time of the month; and in the second half of the month, luteinising hormone

Hysterectomy The operation to remove the womb. There are several ways in which this operation can be performed

Hysteroscopy is the inspection of the inside of the womb using a miniature telescope with a light passing through it

Laparoscopy Inspection of the inside of the abdomen and pelvis using a small telescope

Laparoscopic surgery (Keyhole surgery) Carried out by using thin instruments inserted through the same hole as the laparoscope is passed in to the abdomen and one, two or more holes in the wall of the abdomen

Libido Sex drive

Luteinising hormone Produced by the pituitary gland and acts mainly on the ovary in the second half of the cycle to make it produce progesterone

Menarche The start of the periods. In the UK usually between 12 and 13 years of age but any time between 10 to 16 years is normal. The word is derived from the Latin Mensis = month, Archeos = Greek for the beginning

Menopause The time when the periods stop (from Mensis Latin for month and Pause in the Greek word to cease)

Oestrogen Hormone made in the ovary which acts to thicken the endometrium (see entry). It also acts on the breasts and has some effect on women's moods. There are several different oestrogens made each month by the ovaries

Osteoporosis is a condition in which the bones of the body become weakened because they lose some of their mineral content. The word is derived from three Greek words osteon = bone, poros = passage, osis = condition, so osteoporosis is the condition of the loss of some bone structure

Ovaries are organs the size of walnuts situated beside the uterus in a woman's pelvis. In them ova (eggs) are stored to be released one each month during a woman's reproductive life. The ovaries make two hormones, oestrogens and progesterone

Perimenopausal years The two or three years before the menopause and two or three years after (peri = around)

Premature menopause Menopause occurring earlier than the age of 35

Progesterone Hormone mainly made in the second half of the menstrual cycle by the ovary. It changes the endometrium which has been thickened by oestrogen in to a bed or nest suitable for receiving a fertilised egg. It also can affect women's moods

Progestogen Substance that acts like progesterone

Puberty Beginning of reproductive life for a woman and is characterised by bust development, under arm and pubic hair growth, changes in the shape of the womb so that the upper part becomes bigger and the change in the distribution of body fat

Reproductive life Usually lasts from the age of 15 or a little earlier, or later, until the age of 45. During these thirty years or so a woman is capable of having babies

Uterus Womb

Zoladex (Goserelin) is an analogue, ie a copy, of releasing hormones produced by the hypothalamus. It is used to bring about a short acting medical artificial menopause - primarily to treat endometriosis and to shrink fibroids before they are removed. This preparation effectively stops periods because it shuts off the production of FSH and LH. It cannot be used for a long time

(ii) Useful Addresses

Most large district general hospitals and almost all teaching hospitals in the UK have special clinics for the menopause. The secretary of the gynaecological department in all these hospitals will be able to indicate the hours at which such clinics are held.

✩ **The Amarant Trust**
11 - 13 Charterhouse Buildings, London ECIM 7AN. They have lists of addresses of centres.

✩ **The Amarant Centre in the Churchill Clinic**
80 Lambeth Road, London SE 1 7PW

✩ **The British Homoeopathic Association**
27a Devonshire Street, London WI

✩ **The Homoeopathic Society**
2 Powis Place, London WC1

✩ **Homoeopathy For a Change**
15a St George's Mews, London NWI

✩ **The National Osteoporosis Society**
PO Box 10, Radstock, Bath BA3 3YB. Tel **01761 471771** Fax **01761 471104**

✩ **Wellbeing**
The Royal College of Obstetricians and Gynaecologists, 27 Sussex Place, London NW1. They publish a guide for women's health entitled *Wellbeing of Women* at £7.95 including a £2.00 donation to Wellbeing

(iii) Further Reading

✩ **Understanding HRT and the Menopause**
Which? Consumer Guide (Penguin)

- ☼ **Homoeopathy for the Menopause**
  Dr Trevor Smith (Insight Publishing)
- ☼ **The Menopause**
  Miriam Stoppard (Dorling Kindersley Publishers)
- ☼ **Passage to Power - Natural Menopause Revolution**
  Leslie Kenton (Vermilion Press)

Index

Need2Know Series

For further details and to order further copies, please contact

Kerrie Pateman (Editorial)
Pat Wilson (Marketing)
Need2Know
1-2 Wainman Road
Woodston
Peterborough
Cambs
PE2 7BU

Tel 01733 390801
Fax 01733 230751

Need2Know are always interested in proposals for new titles.
Please contact the above address for information and brief.

Also Published by

Need2Know

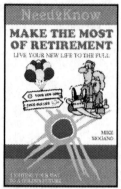

Make the Most of Retirement
Live your New Life to the Full

Mike Mogano
ISBN 1 86144-003-0
£5.99 166pp Pub Jan 96

Aimed at over 10 million pensioners in the UK.

50-75 year olds own 80% of Britain's wealth - accounting for 30% of all consumer expenditure...

Easy to read and packed with ideas and information, *Make the Most of Retirement* is an accessible guide to enjoying the retirement years.

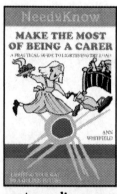

Make the Most of Being a Carer
A Practical Guide to Lightening the Load

Ann Whitfield
ISBN 1 86144-002-2
£5.99 170pp Pub Jan 96

There are around 7 million people who have taken on the role of carer in Britain today. They are mothers, fathers, sons, daughters, grandparents, uncles, aunts...ordinary people in difficult situations.

Practical and detailed, the book covers a wide range of issues.

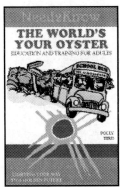

The World's Your Oyster

Education and Learning for Adults

Polly Bird
ISBN 1 86144-014-6
£5.99 110pp Pub July 96

A complete guide to education and training for adults.

The number of mature entrants to higher education in the UK in 1993 was up by 128% on 1982.

Order Information

All Need2Know titles can be ordered through your local bookshop or direct from the publisher.

Payment Details

Please make cheques or postal orders payable to *Forward Press Ltd* adding £1 for postage and packing (if you are ordering more than three copies, postage and packing is free).

Please send orders to:

Distribution, Forward Press Ltd, 1-2 Wainman Road, Woodston, Peterborough PE2 7BU Tel: 01733 238140 Fax: 01733 230751

If you have any order queries please contact the above address.